Special & Tasty Mediterranean Diet Cookbook

Eat Healthy & Lose Weight

Joseph Bellisario

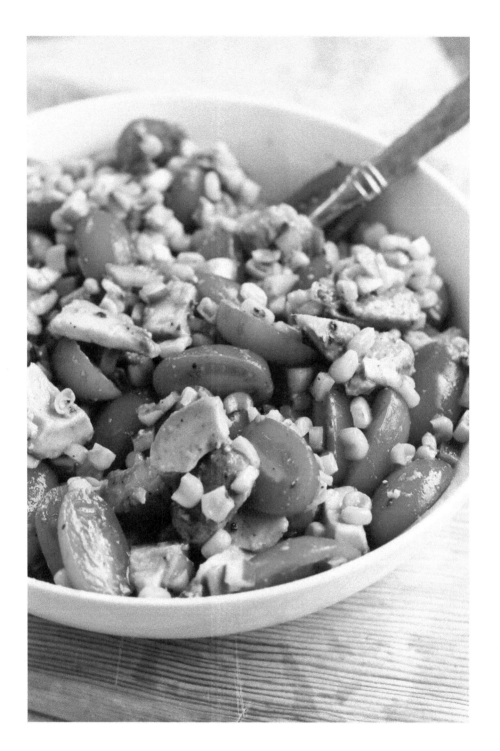

TABLE OF CONTENTS

Blood orange and avocado salad

A combination of oranges and avocado is a nutritional blast for brightening yup one's winter days.

It is packed with seasonal flavors to tease your taste buds.

Ingredients

- ¼ cup of fresh cilantro leaves
- Flaky sea salt
- ¼ small red onion
- 4 blood oranges
- 1 teaspoon of nigella seed, black sesame seeds
- 2 tablespoons of extra virgin olive oil
- 1 large ripe avocado, thinly sliced
- 2 tablespoons of fresh lime juice

Directions

1. Soak the onions for 20 minutes or so in iced water to crisp and softens their flavor intensity.
2. On a large serving plate, layer the orange and avocado slices.

3. Drain the onion and tuck pieces in between and on top of the orange and avocado.
4. Drizzle the salad with the lime juice.
5. Sprinkle with salt.
6. Sprinkle the seeds and cilantro on top.
7. Drizzle with olive oil all over it.
8. Serve and enjoy.

Simple seedy slaw

The simple seedy slaw utilizes a simple lemon dressing to spike up the taste and flavor toasted with pumpkin seeds and sunflower.

It is gluten free perfect for a vegan and Mediterranean Sea diet.

Ingredients

- 1 clove garlic, pressed
- 2 cups of sliced purple cabbage
- ½ teaspoon of ground cumin
- 2 cups of finely sliced green cabbage
- ½ teaspoon of salt
- 2 cups of shredded carrots
- ¼ cup of chopped fresh parsley
- ¾ cup of mixed seeds
- ¼ cup of olive oil
- 3 tablespoons of lemon juice

Directions

1. In a medium serving bowl, combine the prepared purple together with the green cabbage, carrots, and parsley. Set aside.

2. Toast seeds over medium heat, stirring frequently, until the seeds are fragrant.

3. Pour the toasted seeds into the mixing bowl and toss to combine.

4. In a small bowl, combine the olive oil together with 2 tablespoons of lemon juice.

5. Then, add the garlic with cumin and salt, whisk until blended.

6. Drizzle the dressing over the slaw, toss until ingredients are coated in dressing.

7. Serve and enjoy.

Hearty sweet potatoes, arugula, and wild rice salad with ginger dressing

Ingredients

- 1 tablespoon of maple syrup or honey
- 1 cup of wild rice, rinsed
- Fine sea salt, divided
- 2 teaspoons of finely grated fresh ginger
- 1 ½ pounds of sweet potatoes
- 2 tablespoons of apple cider vinegar
- Extra virgin olive oil
- ¾ cup of raw pepitas
- 20 twists of freshly ground black pepper
- 2 tablespoons of Dijon mustard
- ¼ cup of dried cranberries
- 5 ounces of arugula
- ½ cup of crumbled feta
- ½ cup of thinly sliced green onion

Directions

1. Preheat the oven to 425°F.

11

2. Line a large baking sheet with parchment paper.

3. Bring a large pot of water to boil.

4. Once boiling, add rice and continue boiling

5. Lower heat as necessary to prevent overflow, for 55 minutes.

6. Remove, drain any excess water, return the rice to pot.

7. Cover, let rest for 10 minutes, then stir in ¼ teaspoon of the salt.

8. Place the cubed sweet potato on the pan.

9. Drizzle with the olive oil and sprinkle with ¼ teaspoon of the salt. Toss to coat in oil.

10. Arrange the sweet potatoes in a single layer, roast for 30 minutes in the preheated oven, tossing halfway, until tender.

11. Combine extra virgin olive oil, apple cider vinegar, Dijon mustard, maple syrup, ginger, sea salt, and black pepper in a small bowl and whisk until combined. Set aside.

12. Combine the arugula with wild rice and roasted sweet potatoes in a large serving bowl.

13. Spread the seeds on your parchment-covered baking sheet.

14. Bake for 4 minutes, until lightly golden.

15. Spread the toasted seeds.

16. Top with the crumbled feta, green onion, and dried cranberries.

17. Serve and enjoy.

Pomegranate and pear salad with ginger dressing

Ginger is the main flavor in the pomegranate and pear salad recipe.

It features vegetables and herbs for a perfect Mediterranean Sea diet.

Ingredients

- 1 tablespoon of maple syrup
- ½ cup of raw pecans
- 5 ounces of baby arugula
- 1 tablespoon of apple cider vinegar
- ¼ teaspoon of fine sea salt
- 10 twists of freshly ground black pepper
- 2 ounces of goat cheese
- 1 tablespoon of Dijon mustard
- 1 large ripe Bartlett pear
- 1 honey crisp
- 1 teaspoon of finely grated fresh ginger
- Arils from 1 pomegranate
- ¼ cup of extra virgin olive oil

Directions

1. Place the pecans in a skillet over medium heat.
2. Toast, stirring often, until fragrant for 5 minutes or so.
3. Remove, and roughly chop. Set aside.
4. Arrange the arugula across a large serving platter.
5. Sprinkle the chopped pecans and crumbled goat cheese over the arugula.
6. Arrange slices of pear and apple across the salad in sections.
7. Then, sprinkle all over with fresh pomegranate arils.
8. Combine extra virgin olive oil, apple cider vinegar, Dijon mustard, maple syrup, ginger, sea salt, and black pepper, whisk until blended.
9. Taste, and adjust the seasoning.
10. Drizzle the ginger dressing lightly all over the salad.
11. Serve and enjoy.

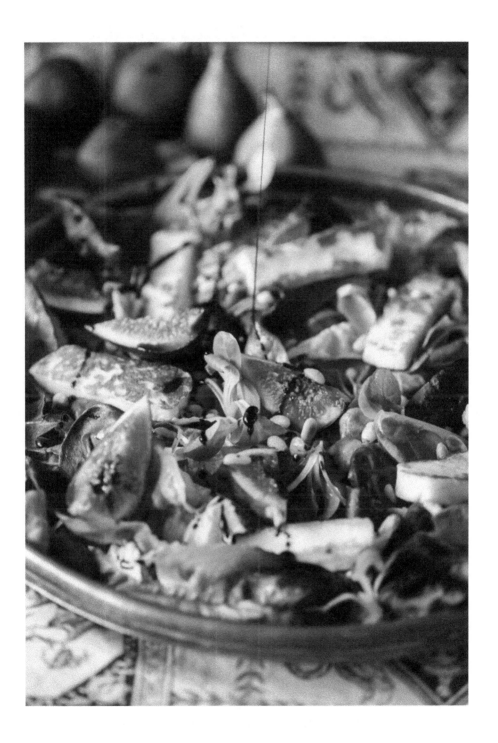

Wild rice and kale salad

Ingredients

- 1 cup of cherry tomatoes
- 5 green onions
- 1 cup of wild rice
- 1 ¼ cups of water
- 2 tablespoons of extra virgin olive oil
- 1 medium red bell pepper
- 1 small of bunch kale
- ½ cup of crumbled feta cheese
- ¼ cup of lemon juice
- 1 clove garlic, pressed
- ½ teaspoon of fine sea salt
- ¼ teaspoon of ground black pepper
- 2 teaspoons of maple syrup

Directions

1. Add the wild rice and water to an Instant Pot.
2. Secure the lid and move the steam release valve to Sealing.
3. Cook on high pressure for 22 minutes.
4. Whisk together the olive oil, lemon juice, garlic, salt, pepper, and maple syrup for the dressing. Set aside.

5. Add chopped kale, green onions, red bell pepper, and tomatoes to the bowl.

6. Toss the vegetables to coat.

7. When the cooking cycle is complete, let the pressure naturally release for 10 minutes, then move the steam release valve to Venting to release any remaining pressure.

8. When the floating valve drops, remove the lid and give the rice a stir.

9. Add the rice to the bowl of dressed vegetables.

10. Taste and adjust the seasoning.

11. Serve and enjoy.

Fresh mint dressing

Mint is as fresh as it feels in the mouth.

This delicious mint dressing recipe features lemon juice and natural honey for better taste that suits a Mediterranean style.

Ingredients

- 2 cloves garlic, roughly chopped
- ½ cup of extra virgin olive oil
- ¼ teaspoon of sea salt
- ½ cup of lemon juice
- ¼ cup of packed fresh mint leaves
- 10 twists of freshly ground black pepper
- 3 tablespoons of honey
- 1 tablespoon of Dijon mustard

Directions

1. In a food processor, combine all of the above ingredients and blend until smooth.
2. Taste, and adjust the seasoning accordingly.
3. Serve and enjoy.
4. Any leftover should be refrigerated for up to 1 week.

Fattoush salad with mint dressing

Ingredients

- ½ cup of chopped radish
- 2 whole grain pitas
- ½ cup of torn fresh mint leaves
- 2 tablespoons of extra virgin olive oil
- ½ cup of crumbled feta
- 1 cup of chopped red onion
- Pinch of fine sea salt
- ½ batch of fresh mint dressing
- Ground sumac
- 10 ounces of fresh romaine lettuce
- 1 large tomato, chopped
- 1 cup of quartered and thinly sliced Persian cucumber

Directions

1. Preheat your oven to 400°F.
2. Toss the torn pita with 2 tablespoons olive oil until lightly coated.
3. Sprinkle with salt, bake in the oven until the pieces golden in 12 minutes, tossing halfway.

4. Let to cool.

5. In a large serving bowl, combine the chopped lettuce together with the tomatoes, cucumber, parsley, onion, radish, mint, and feta, and toasted pita.

6. Drizzle with ½ cup of the dressing over the salad.

7. Gently toss to lightly coated in dressing.

8. Serve and enjoy sprinkled with sumac.

Fresh herbed avocado salad

Variety of herb mix is used to cover the avocado with lime honey dressing and toasted pepitas.

It is as healthy as any other Mediterranean Sea diet recipe.

Ingredients

- 2 teaspoons honey or maple syrup
- ½ cup raw pepitas
- Extra virgin olive oil
- ¼ teaspoon chili powder
- ½ teaspoon fine sea salt
- Pinch of salt
- ½ chopped radish
- ½ cup chopped green onion
- ¼ cup lime juice
- Lime zest for garnish
- ½ cup chopped fresh cilantro, parsley, basil, dill
- 1 medium jalapeño
- 4 large just-ripe avocados

Directions

1. Toast the pepitas in a large skillet over medium heat, stirring often, until golden on the edges.
2. Remove, stir in the chili powder together with the olive oil and pinch of salt. Let cool.
3. In a mixing dish, combine the chopped radish, green onion, herbs and jalapeño. Set aside.
4. Then, whisk together the lime juice, olive oil, honey, and salt in a small bowl. Set aside.
5. Place the avocado in a medium serving bowl.
6. Drizzle the dressing all over it.
7. Stir the toasted pepitas into the herb mix, then spoon it over the avocados.
8. Serve and enjoy.

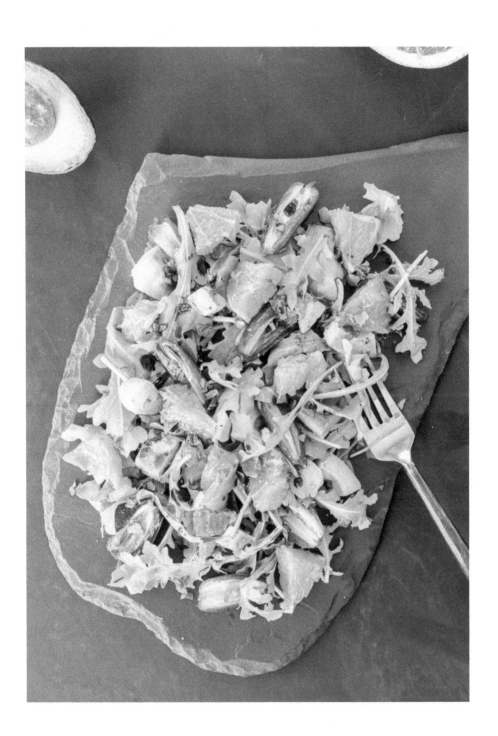

Sliced fennel, orange and almond salad

Ingredients

- Sherry vinegar
- 3 bulbs of fennel
- Extra virgin olive oil
- 1 handful of almonds
- 2 handfuls of rocket
- 3 oranges
- A few springs of fresh mint

Directions

1. Peeler and place the fennel in a bowl of ice water.
2. Toast the almonds in a dry frying pan, crush in a pestle.
3. Arranged slice the oranges on a platter.
4. Drain the fennel, mix together with the mint, rocket, a splash of sherry vinegar and oil.
5. Season with sea salt and black pepper
6. Scatter the fennel mixture over the oranges topping with toasted almonds.
7. Serve and enjoy.

Roasted squash and couscous salad

Ingredients

- 2 tablespoons of pumpkin seeds
- 1 butternut squash
- 1 fresh green chili
- ½ of a lemon
- 5 sprigs of fresh thyme
- 100g of couscous
- 1 tablespoon cumin seeds
- Olive oil

Directions

1. Preheat the oven to 375°F.
2. Place the squash and chili into a roasting dish.
3. Spread over the cumin seeds together with thyme sprigs, and olive oil.
4. Season with sea salt.
5. Let roast for 50 minutes, or until lightly golden, turning halfway.
6. Place the couscous in a bowl, add enough boiling water above the couscous.

7. Cover the bowl and leave for 10 minutes.

8. Toast the pumpkin seeds in a dry frying pan.

9. Stir in the lemon zest and juice, roasted squash and olive oil.

10. Serve and enjoy wit scattered pumpkin seeds.

Spicy cucumber pickle

Ingredients

- 150ml of vinegar
- 2 banana shallots
- 2-star anise
- 2 teaspoons of mustard seeds
- 6 pickling cucumbers
- ½ teaspoon of ground turmeric
- 75g of caster sugar

Directions

1. Place the cucumbers together with the shallots in a colander.
2. Sprinkle with 2 teaspoons of sea salt.
3. Rinse after 45 minutes.
4. Combine all the other ingredients in a pan let boil.
5. Stir until the sugar dissolves.
6. Fit the cucumbers snugly into a jar.
7. Pour over the liquid.
8. Seal and leave for 24 hours.
9. Serve and enjoy.

Spicy feta and pepper dip

Ingredients

- 3 tablespoons of olive oil
- 240g of feta cheese
- 120g of jarred red peppers

Directions

1. Combine the feta, olive oil, and red pepper in a blender.
2. Season with black pepper, then blend until smooth.
3. Transfer to a serving bowl.
4. Serve and enjoy.

Seafood Mediterranean recipes

Amongst the various Mediterranean Sea diets, seafood particularly has a gigantic amount of protein significant for muscle building.

The seafood includes crabs, oyster, fish, sardines, trout, salmon, mussels, and clams, which can feature coconut milk, lime, lemon, jalapeno, cinnamon, garlic, onions, ginger, apple, lentil, lettuce, and many more other vegetables and fruits including whole foods.

The seafood recipe includes;

Brazilian fish stew (Moqueca)

This incredible Mediterranean fish stew features coconut milk with lime and jalapeno with favorite flavors perfect for any meal.

Ingredients

- 1 teaspoon of salt
- ½ cup chopped cilantro, scallions
- 1 lime- zest and juice
- 3 tablespoons of coconut
- 1 14 ounce can of coconut milk
- 1 cup of fish or chicken stock
- 1 onion- finely diced
- 1 pounds of firm white fish- Halibut
- 2 teaspoons of paprika
- 1 cup of carrot, diced
- 1 red bell pepper, diced
- Squeeze of lime
- 4 garlic cloves- rough chopped
- ½ jalapeno, finely diced
- 1 tablespoon of tomato paste
- 1 teaspoon of ground cumin
- 1 cups of tomatoes, diced

Directions

1. Place pat dry fish cut in pieces in a bowl.
2. Add salt together with the zest from half the lime and lime juice massage to coat. Set aside.
3. In a large pan, heat the olive oil over medium heat.
4. Then, add onion together with salt , let sauté 3 minutes.
5. Lower the heat, add carrot with bell pepper, garlic, and jalapeno.
6. Allow to cook for 5 minutes.
7. Add tomato paste with the spices and stock.
8. Mix and let simmer, then add tomatoes.
9. Cover, continue to simmer over low heat for 5 minutes.
10. Add the coconut milk and season accordingly.
11. Nestle the fish in the stew and simmer until cooked through in6 minutes.
12. Spoon the flavorful coconut broth over the fish cook until desired.
13. Taste and adjust accordingly.
14. Serve and enjoy with rice.

Simple salmon chowder

Ingredients

- 1/3 cup of vermouth
- 3 tablespoons of olive oil
- Fennel fronds, lemon wedges, fresh dill
- 1 onion, diced
- 3 cups of fish or chicken stock
- 1 teaspoon of salt
- 1 small fennel bulb,
- 1 lb. salmon, skinless
- 1 cup of celery, sliced
- 2 cups of whole milk
- 4 garlic cloves, rough chopped
- 1 teaspoon of fennel seeds
- ½ teaspoon of thyme
- ½ teaspoon of smoked paprika
- ¾ lb. of baby potatoes, thinly sliced
- 1 bay leaf

Directions

1. Start by heating olive oil over medium heat.
2. Sauté the onion with fennel and celery for 6 minutes.

3. Add garlic with fennel seeds , thyme, and sauté again briefly, stirring.

4. Add the smoked paprika .

5. Add vermouth let cook for 2 minutes.

6. Then, add the stock together with the salt , thyme and bay, simmer over high heat.

7. Add potatoes and stir.

8. Cover, bring to a simmer over low heat until tender in 10 minutes

9. Add the milk and bring to a low simmer.

10. Add the salmon, poach in the soup for 2 minutes.

11. Taste, and adjust seasonings accordingly.

12. Serve and enjoy garnished with fennel fronds, lemon wedges, and or fresh dill.

Furikake salmon bowls

This furikake salmon bowls are a delicious Mediterranean Sea diet fish recipe elevated by the shiitake mushrooms, avocado, and cabbage.

Ingredients

1. 2 extra-large handfuls of shredded cabbage
2. 10 ounces of salmon
3. 4 ounces of shiitake mushrooms
4. Scallions, furikake , cucumber, chili flakes
5. 3 tablespoons of soy sauce
6. 3 tablespoons of Mirin
7. 2 tablespoons of sesame oil
8. 1 tablespoon of Furikake
9. 2 cups of cooked rice
10. Pinch of salt , pepper and chili flakes
11. 1 avocado , sliced

Directions

1. Cook rice according to the package Directions.
2. Mix soy sauce together with the mirin in a small bowl.

3. Then, heat the sesame oil in a large skillet over medium high heat.
4. Season with a pinch of salt , pepper and chili flakes.
5. Add the salmon with mushrooms, and sear all sides, until turns golden.
6. Turn off the heat let cool slightly.
7. Spoon sauce over top of the salmon and mushrooms, swirling the skillet. Keep aside for later.
8. Divide rice between 2 bowls.
9. Sprinkle with furikake .
10. Organize the cabbage and avocado wedges in the bowl.
11. Top with seared salmon and mushrooms.
12. Sprinkle with Furikake and the remaining sauce over the avocado and cabbage.
13. Serve and enjoy immediately.

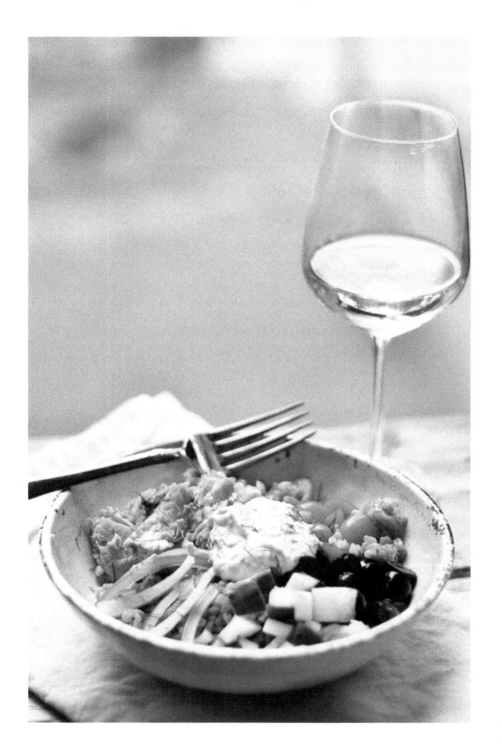

Lemony zucchini noodles with halibut

Ingredients

- 16 ounces of zucchini noodles
- 1 garlic clove, smashed
- Sweet cherry tomatoes, chili flakes, optional
- 2 tablespoons of olive oil
- 2 teaspoons lemon zest
- Salt and pepper to taste
- ½ cup chopped Italian parsley
- 10 ounces of halibut
- 1 tablespoon of olive oil
- 1 fat shallot, sliced thin
- 3 garlic cloves, rough chopped
- 1 tablespoon lemon juice

Directions

1. Preheat your oven ready to 375F.
2. Heat oil in a medium skillet over medium heat.
3. When hot enough, add smashed garlic clove and swirl to infuse.

4. Pat fish dry and season with salt and pepper searing both sides until golden.

5. Place in the warm oven until cooked through in 6 minutes.

6. In a large skillet, heat another oil over medium heat.

7. Add shallots together with the garlic, stirring until fragrant in 3 minutes.

8. Then, add the zucchini noodles, season with salt and pepper.

9. Sauté until noodles for 4 minutes.

10. Toss in lemon zest, fresh parsley, and a squeeze of lemon.

11. Taste, and adjust accordingly.

12. Divide among two bowls and top with the halibut.

13. Serve and enjoy.

Spicy miso ramen with chili roasted salmon and bok choy

This recipe is perfect for a vegan and Mediterranean Sea diet.

It draws it distinction from the mushrooms, scallions, roasted chili and paleo.

Ingredients

- 3 scallions
- 6 ounces of salmon, thinly sliced
- 4 ounces of shitake mushrooms
- 4 ounces of fresh ramen noodles
- 2 tablespoons of soy sauce
- 2 baby bok choy – sliced, lengthwise
- 2 teaspoons of honey or maple
- 3 teaspoons of garlic chili paste
- 4 cups of chicken broth
- 2 tablespoons of miso paste
- ½ teaspoon of hondashi granules
- 1 tablespoon of toasted sesame oil

Directions

1. Preheat your oven ready to 400 F.
2. Stir the soy sauce together with the honey , sesame oil , and chili paste in a small bowl.
3. Brush the marinade over both sides of salmon and shitakes.
4. Place on a parchment lined baking sheet.
5. Let broil for 5 minutes, set aside.
6. Bring the stock to a simmer in a medium pot .
7. Add miso with hondashi, stir until combined.
8. Add the bok choy and scallions, let wilt.
9. Lower heat let simmer.
10. Taste, and adjust seasoning accordingly.
11. Divide the noodles among two bowls.
12. Top with the salmon and shitakes.
13. Organize the bok choy around the noodles, ladling the flavorful broth on top.
14. Garnish with fresh scallions or crispy shallots
15. Serve and enjoy.

Wood-fired shellfish

Ingredients

- Extra virgin olive oil
- 2 kg of mixed seafood
- 2 lemons
- Freshly ground black pepper
- 2 cloves garlic, peeled
- A few sprigs of soft fresh herbs
- Sea salt

Directions

1. Start by firing up your wood-fired oven ready to 380°F.
2. Clean and wash the shellfish, pulling the beards off the mussels, discard any open ones.
3. Bash the garlic with a good pinch of sea salt in a pestle and mortar until creamy, then grate in the lemon zest.
4. Add a good pinch of black pepper with enough extra virgin olive oil to make a dressing.
5. Place the shellfish into a large roasting tray.
6. Drizzle with the dressing, toss together.
7. Spread the shellfish out into an even layer.
8. Add halved lemon to the tray, slide into the hot oven, roast for 10 minutes.

9. Serve and enjoy with herb leaves.

Smoky barbecue shellfish

Ingredients

- 2kg of shellfish
- 2 handfuls of fresh flat-leaf parsley
- 1 clove of garlic
- Herb branches
- 3 lemons
- 4 fresh red chilies
- Extra virgin olive oil

Directions

1. Begin by adding the garlic together with the lemon zest and juice to a large bowl.
2. Pour in 3 times the amount of extra virgin olive oil with finely chopped parsley stalks. Mix.
3. Smoke the herb branches on the Barbie.
4. Drain the shellfish, throw onto the hottest part of the Barbie.
5. Lift the sides up after 3 minutes to check the shellfish have opened.
6. Remove them to the dressing bowl, remove out any shellfish that have not opened.

7. Sprinkle over many chopped parsley and chili, mix together.
8. Serve and enjoy.

Garlic prawn kebabs

Ingredients

1. 20g feta cheese
2. Olive oil
3. 75g of sourdough bread
4. Extra virgin olive oil
5. 1 lemon
6. 160g of raw peeled king prawns
7. 1 x 400g tin of cherry tomatoes
8. ½ x 460g jar of roasted red peppers
9. 3 cloves of garlic
10. ½ a bunch of flat-leaf parsley

Directions

1. Preheat the grill to high.
2. Slice and cut the bread into 3cm chunks, place in a large bowl with the prawns, sliced peppers, garlic, parsley, half of lemon juice, olive oil, a pinch of black pepper, and stalk. Mix well.
3. Skewer up the prawns and bread on 2 skewers, interlacing with the peppers.
4. Sit each skewer across a roasting tray, grilling for 8 minutes, turning halfway.

5. Place a non-stick frying pan on a medium heat.

6. Add ½ a tablespoon of olive oil and the sliced garlic, stir regularly for 2 minutes.

7. Pour in the tinned tomatoes to bubble away until the skewers are ready.

8. Add a squeeze of lemon juice, then season the sauce to taste.

9. Serve the kebabs on top of the sauce, sprinkled with feta and black pepper.

10. Serve and enjoy with extra virgin olive oil.

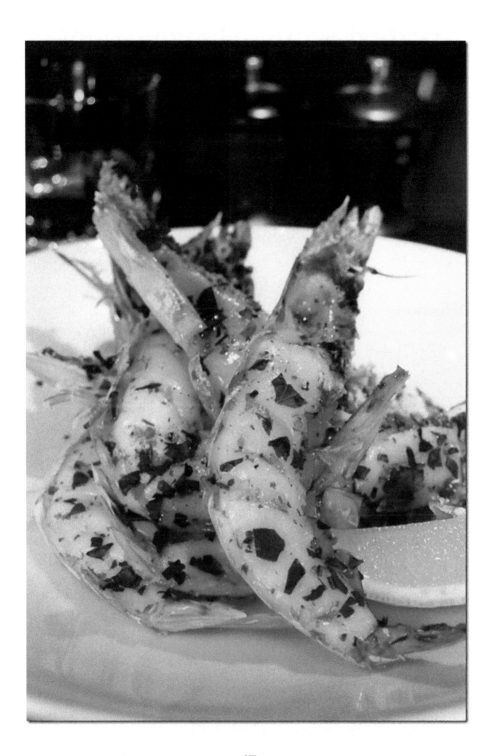

Grilled Scottish langoustines

Ingredients

- 40g of unsalted butter
- 10 medium langoustines
- 1 lemon
- 25g of 'nduja

Directions

1. Add 40g sea salt to 2 liters of water, bring to a boil in a large pan.
2. Have a large bowl ready with 2 liters of ice-cold water.
3. Plunge the langoustines into the boiling water briefly, remove and refresh in the cold water, let dry.
4. Preheat the grill to medium high heat.
5. In a blender, process the 'nduja with 20ml of warm water until smooth.
6. Add the butter, blend to combine.
7. Lay the langoustines cut-side-up on a large roasting tray, loosen them within their shells, and spoon over the 'nduja butter.
8. Transfer Place under the grill until the butter is bubbling and the langoustines are golden.
9. Finish with a squeeze of lemon juice.

10. Serve and enjoy.

Baked clams with roasted sweet shallots and fennel

Ingredients

- 300ml of Italian white wine
- 1 large bulb of fennel
- 1 lemon
- 1 bunch of fresh flat-leaf parsley
- 1 teaspoon of fennel seeds
- 20 round shallots
- 1 teaspoon of dried chili flakes
- Olive oil
- 1.8kg of large Italian clams

Directions

1. Preheat the oven to 350°F.
2. Place the shallots with cut-side-up in a large roasting tray.
3. Add fennel wedges to the tray.
4. Bash fennel seeds with chili flakes in a pestle and mortar, then sprinkle over the shallots.
5. Drizzle over 4 tablespoons of olive oil, season.

6. Let bake in the oven for 25 minutes, or until the shallots are golden.

7. Remove the shallots and fennel from the oven.

8. Raise the heat to the maximum.

9. Add the clams to the tray of juices and pour over the wine.

10. Pick and finely chop the parsley, grate the lemon zest, mix most of it through.

11. Rub the halved lemon with olive oil, then place in the pan, then cover the dish with tin foil.

12. Let bake for 15 minutes.

13. Sprinkle the remaining lemon zest and parsley over the dish and gently fold everything through the cooking juices.

14. Serve and enjoy with chilled Italian wine and crusty bread.

Sizzling seared scallops

Ingredients

- 8 raw king scallops
- 200g of frozen peas
- 50g of firm black pudding
- 400g of potatoes
- ½ a bunch of fresh mint

Directions

1. Cook chopped potatoes in a pan of boiling salted water for 12 minutes.
2. Add the peas for the last 3 minutes.
3. Place a non-stick frying pan on a medium high heat.
4. Place 1 tablespoon of olive oil once hot, with the remaining mint leaves in to crisp briefly.
5. Then, scoop the leaves on to a plate, leave the olive oil in the pan.
6. Season the scallops with sea salt and black pepper.
7. Let fry for 2 minutes on each side, or until golden.
8. Crumble in the black pudding.
9. Drain the peas with the potatoes, then, return to the pan, mash with the chopped mint and 1 tablespoon of extra virgin olive oil.

10. Taste, and adjust the seasoning.

11. Serve and enjoy drizzled with extra virgin olive oil and sprinkle over the crispy mint.

Beetroot curry

What a blessing to add onto your body blood. Beet root is a gift to replenish blood in the body; as such, this recipe cannot be underestimated among Mediterranean Sea diets with earthly flavors.

Ingredients

- 1 teaspoon of hot curry powder
- 3 cloves of garlic
- 2 tablespoons of desiccated coconut
- 3 cloves of garlic
- 5cm of piece of ginger
- vegetable oil
- 2 teaspoons of black mustard seeds
- 1 kg mixed beets
- 250g of ripe cherry tomatoes
- 7g of dried curry leaves
- ½ a bunch of fresh coriander
- 320g of wild rice
- 6 spring onions
- 14g of dried curry leaves
- 5cm of piece of ginger
- 1 x 400ml tin of light coconut milk

- 1 lemon
- 1 lime
- 2 fresh long red chilies

Directions

1. Place a large pan over a medium heat.
2. Add the curry leaves with the curry powder, mustard seeds, and coconut, let toast for 2 minute. Transfer to a food processor and blend well.
3. Add spring onions to the food processor with garlic, ginger, and vegetable oil.
4. Pulse to forms a paste.
5. Place the pan back on the hob over a medium heat.
6. Add the paste cook briefly, add beetroot.
7. Lower heat and cook until sticky and gnarly, stirring often.
8. Add the cherry tomatoes and cook for 5 minutes, then break them with the back of a spoon.
9. Cook the rice as instructed on the packet.
10. Stir in the coconut milk with a squeeze of lemon juice.
11. Raise the heat let cook for 5 minutes.
12. Season to taste.
13. Place a frying pan over a medium heat with oil.
14. Add all the temper ingredients let heat for 2 minutes.

15. Turn off the heat, transfer into a bowl lined with kitchen paper.
16. Serve the curry with the rice and temper and or coriander leaves scattered on top.
17. Serve and enjoy.

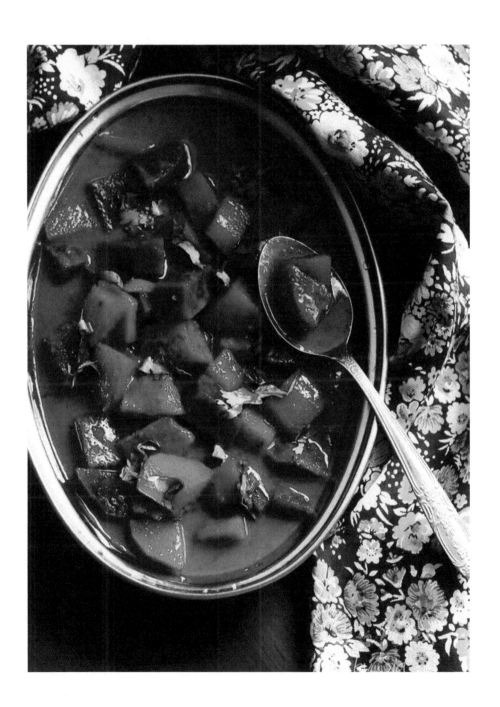

Brick lane burger

Everyone likes to enjoy a delicious burger, isn't it?

If yes, then this Mediterranean Sea diet recipe is a must try for you.

It has great flavors derived from onions, garlic and ginger.

Ingredients

- 200g of butternut squash
- 2 cloves of garlic
- 2 fresh green chilies
- 100g of paneer cheese
- Mango chutney
- 1 big bunch of fresh coriander
- 150g of gram flour
- 6 burger buns
- 2 teaspoons of ground turmeric
- 3 poppadoms
- 2 baby gem lettuce
- 1 carrot
- 2 teaspoons of ground cumin
- 2 red onions
- 2 limes

- Olive oil
- 100ml of natural yoghurt
- 5cm of piece of ginger
- 1 fresh red chili

Directions

1. Preheat the oven to 350°F.
2. Place onions, carrots, paneer, garlic, ginger, and coriander into a large mixing bowl.
3. Place flour together with the turmeric and cumin.
4. Season with sea salt and black pepper, squeeze in the juice of 1 lime with water, mix with your hands.
5. Divide into 6, then shape and squash into patties.
6. Drizzle with bit of oil into a large non-stick frying pan over a medium heat.
7. Let fry the patties for 3 minutes on each side or until golden.
8. Remove to a baking tray for 10 minutes or until cooked.
9. Pestle the remaining coriander leaves, setting aside a handful.
10. Add a pinch of salt, then bash to a paste. Squeeze in the juice of lime, stir in the yoghurt.
11. Spoon a little coriander yoghurt over the base and inside lid of each burger bun.

12. Crumble the poppadoms, sprinkle over the yoghurt, then sit a patty on top of each base and spread with 1 tablespoon of mango chutney.

13. Top with a handful of lettuce and the reserved coriander leaves.

14. Sprinkle with red chili

15. Serve and enjoy.

Summer vegetable lasagna

Ingredients

- Olive oil
- ½ x 30g tin of anchovies in oil
- 6 cloves of garlic
- 500g of fresh lasagne sheets
- 700g of asparagus
- 1 lemon
- Sprigs of fresh thyme
- 500g of frozen peas
- 300g of frozen broad beans
- Parmesan cheese
- 1 bunch of spring onions
- 1 big bunch of fresh mint
- 300ml of single cream
- 300m of organic vegetable stock
- 2 x 250g tubs of cottage cheese

Directions

1. Preheat the grill to full temperature.
2. Pour oil from the anchovy tin into a large frying pan over a high heat
3. Add the spring onions and anchovies.

4. Add crushed garlic, toss well.

5. Add asparagus stems to the pan, keep tips for later.

6. Season with sea salt and black pepper.

7. Add a splash of boiling water, let cook for a few minutes, stirring occasionally.

8. Add the peas together with the broad beans, mint, lemon zest, and the cream to the pan.

9. Squash, then season with salt and pepper.

10. Pour in the stock and bring to the boil.

11. Stir in 1 tub of cottage cheese.

12. Place a roasting tray over a medium heat.

13. Cover the bottom of the tray with the vegetable mixture, then top with a layer of lasagna sheets, and Parmesan grating.

14. Repeat the layers with the rest of the vegetable mixture and pasta, use lasagne sheets to finish.

15. Mix the remaining tub of cottage cheese with splash of water.

16. Toss the reserved asparagus with a drizzle of oil.

17. Strip over the thyme leaves.

18. Turn the heat under the tray up to high and cook until the lasagne starts to bubble, place under the grill on the middle shelf for 8 minutes.

19. Serve and enjoy.

Gnarly cauliflower curry

Ingredients

- ½ x 400g tin of light coconut milk
- 1 medium cauliflower
- 2 heaped tablespoons of rogan josh curry paste
- Extra virgin olive oil
- 2 heaped tablespoons of natural yoghurt
- 1 red onion
- 1 pinch of dried red chili flakes
- 2 cloves of garlic
- 150g of basmati rice
- 2 lemons
- 4 uncooked poppadoms
- ½ a bunch of fresh coriander
- Pickled chilies

Directions

1. Preheat the grill to high.
2. Place prepared cauliflower in a large pan.
3. Rub the cauliflower with Rogan josh paste.
4. Season with sea salt and black pepper.
5. Add in the cauliflower leaves then place over a medium heat on the hob with water.

6. Add in the garlic, onions, on top of the cauliflower.

7. Bring to the boil, let bubble for 10 minutes.

8. Transfer the pan to the grill, 5cm away, for 15 minutes or until gnarly, charred and cooked through.

9. Cook the rice in a pan of boiling salted water per the packet instruction with half a lemon, drain excess water.

10. Pick the coriander leaves from 1 sprig and scatter over with a few pickled chilies and liquor. Mix.

11. Drizzle with 1 tablespoon of oil.

12. Remove the cauliflower, place over a medium heat.

13. Pour in the coconut milk let boil, stirring gently.

14. One-by-one, puff up your dry poppadoms in the microwave briefly.

15. Add coriander stalks to a pestle with a pinch of salt and chili flakes blend to a paste.

16. Muddle in the yoghurt.

17. Sprinkle the coriander leaves over the curry, add lemon into rice.

18. Serve and enjoy with poppadoms, and lemon pickle.

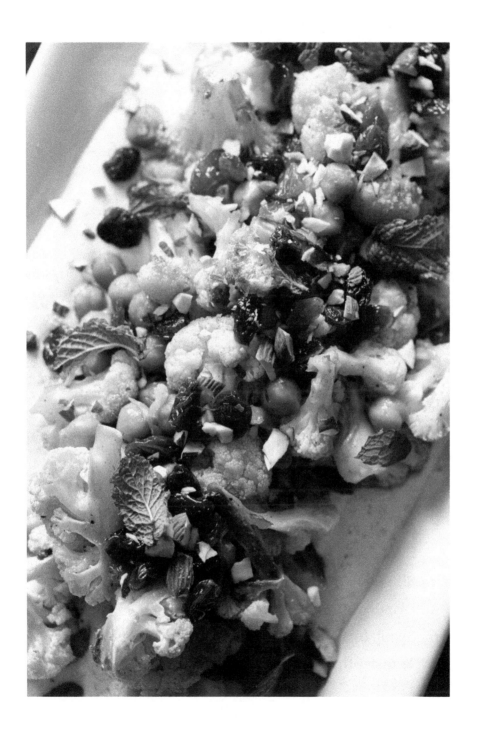

Pot roasted cauliflower

Ingredients

- 1 small pinch of saffron
- Olive oil
- 1 large head of cauliflower
- 6 cloves of garlic
- 3 onions
- 6 large green olives
- 6 anchovy fillets in oil
- 500ml of white wine

Directions

1. Preheat the oven to 350°F.
2. Combine onions, olive oil, and anchovies in an ovenproof pan on a medium-high heat.
3. Add olive with the garlic let cook for 2 minutes, pour in the wine with saffron.
4. Sit the cauliflower in the pan, stalk side down.
5. Drizzle with 1 tablespoon of oil.
6. Spoon bit of onions and liquid over the cauliflower, boil.
7. Transfer the pan to the oven for 1 hour.

8. Carefully lift the cauliflower on to a platter and spoon over the soft onions, olives and fragrant juices from the pan.

9. Serve and enjoy with sliced onions and olives.

Peas, beans, chili and mint

Ingredients

- 1 lemon
- 1 fresh red chili
- 200g of fresh podded
- ½ a bunch of fresh mint
- 200g of fresh podded

Directions

1. Put the mint stalks in a pan of boiling salted water, with the beans and peas to cook for 4 minutes.
2. Combine leafy mint, lemon zest, extra virgin oil, and chili in a bowl, mix.
3. Season with sea salt and black pepper.
4. Drain the beans and peas, reserving some cooking water for later.
5. Pinch the skins off any larger beans, pour the beans and peas on to a platter, toss with a few splashes of reserved cooking water, then spoon over the dressing.
6. Drizzle with extra virgin olive oil and toss together.
7. Serve and enjoy.

Dressed beets

This recipe embraces the healthy benefits of beets, citrus, vinegar and walnuts for a perfect Mediterranean Sea diet.

Ingredients

- 100g of crumbly goat's cheese
- 4 clementine
- 600g of raw mixed-color baby beets
- 40g of shelled unsalted walnut halves
- Extra virgin olive oil
- Red wine vinegar
- ½ a bunch of fresh tarragon

Directions

1. Cook the beets covered, in a pan of boiling salted water for 20 minutes.
2. Squeeze the juice of 1 clementine into a large bowl with extra virgin olive oil and red wine vinegar.
3. Slice and arrange remaining clementine on a plates.
4. Drain the beets rub off the skins when cooled under running water.

5. Season with sea salt and black pepper, add the tarragon and toss with the reserved beet leaves.
6. Divide between your plates, crumble over the goat's cheese and walnuts.
7. Serve an enjoy drizzled with extra virgin olive oil.

Roasted roots halloumi tray bake with courgette tangles

Ingredients

- 4 tablespoons of quality green pesto
- 1 small broccoli
- Olive oil
- 800g of mixed root veggies
- 250g of halloumi cheese
- 2 red peppers
- 1 large eating apple
- 1 courgette
- 100g of lamb's lettuce

Directions

1. Preheat the oven to 400°F.
2. Spread the veg out on a large roasting tray.
3. Drizzle with olive oil.
4. Then, season with sea salt and black pepper, toss to coat.
5. Let roast until the vegetables are tender and colored.
6. Cut and scatter over the veggies.
7. Switch the oven to grill, raise the heat and grill for 10 minutes.

8. Spiralize the courgette.

9. Combine sliced apple with the roasted veggies, then stir through the courgetti and spinach.

10. Mix the pesto with 2 tablespoons of oil and drizzle over.

11. Serve and enjoy.

Parsnip beetroot gratin

Ingredients

- 2 oranges
- 500g of beetroots
- 300ml of double cream
- Unsalted butter
- ½ a bunch of fresh rosemary
- 200ml of crème fraiche
- 500g of parsnips
- 4 cloves of garlic

Directions

1. Preheat the oven to 400°F.
2. Oil a 1.5-liter baking dish ready.
3. Layer up sliced parsnips and beets in the baking dish.
4. Put the cream together with the crème fraîche, whole unpeeled garlic, and rosemary sprigs in a saucepan, let simmer.
5. Remove the heat, add orange zest.
6. Season with sea salt and a big pinch of black pepper.
7. Pour the cream over the vegetables, pressing them to submerge in the liquid and arrange the rosemary sprigs on top.

8. Cover tightly with tin foil

9. Let bake for 45 minutes, until the vegetable is almost tender.

10. Remove the foil and continue to bake for 25 minutes.

11. Cool for 5 minutes.

12. Serve and enjoy.

Roasted radish and runner bean tray bake

Ingredients

- 25g of Cheddar cheese
- 1 tablespoon of red wine vinegar
- 150g of runner beans
- 70g of ciabatta
- Sprigs of fresh dill, flat-leaf parsley, chives
- 6 radishes, with tops
- 3 cloves of garlic
- 1 teaspoon of runny honey
- 100ml of white wine
- 2 courgettes
- Olive oil
- Extra virgin olive oil

Directions

1. Preheat the oven to 375°F.
2. Pour in the wine or stock.
3. Season with sea salt and black pepper, drizzle over 2 tablespoons of olive oil.

4. Coarsely blend the cheddar and sprinkle over the bread pieces.
5. Let roast in the oven for 40 minutes or until cooked through.
6. Combine 2 tablespoons of extra virgin olive oil with the honey and vinegar.
7. Stir through the chopped herbs, season and keep aside.
8. Remove the tray from the oven and drizzle with the dressing.
9. Serve and enjoy on a bed of spinach.

Apricot, root veggie cake with honey yogurt icing

Ingredients

- 150g of Greek-style natural yoghurt
- 40g of pumpkin seeds
- 1 beetroot
- 2 parsnips
- 1 orange
- 1 lemon
- 120g of quality maple syrup
- 2 large free-range eggs
- 25g of clear runny honey
- 70 ml cold-pressed rapeseed oil
- 150g of wholegrain spelt flour
- 1 pinch of mixed spice
- 2 medium carrots
- 1 teaspoon baking powder
- 60g of dried apricots
- 150g of cream cheese
- ½ teaspoon of quality vanilla extract

Directions

1. Preheat the oven to 350°F.
2. Oil the base and sides of a loose-bottomed cake tin with a little rapeseed oil.
3. Line the base with baking paper.
4. Grate and combine the carrots, beetroot and parsnip into a large bowl.
5. Add grated zest of the orange and 2/3 to the veggie with maple syrup, eggs, and rapeseed oil.
6. Fold in the flour, spice, baking powder and a pinch of salt.
7. Add diced apricot with seeds to the bowl, Mix to combine.
8. Pour the mixture into the prepared tin let bake for 40 minutes, rotating the tin after 20 minutes.
9. Let cool in the tin.
10. Whisk together all the ingredients except the lemon, until smooth.
11. Squeeze in a tiny bit of lemon juice and whisk again.
12. Chill in the fridge until needed.
13. Transfer to a plate finish with the icing.
14. Slice and enjoy.

Roasted sprouts

Ingredients

- 1 small clove of garlic
- 500g of Brussels sprouts
- 1 lemon
- 25g of hazelnuts
- 2 teaspoons of coriander seeds
- 1 heaped teaspoon of tahini
- 2 small red onions
- ½ a bunch of fresh coriander
- 1 bulb of fennel
- Olive oil
- 1 pinch of sumac
- 1 teaspoon of sesame seeds
- 1 teaspoon of cumin seeds
- 200g of Greek yoghurt

Directions

1. Preheat the oven to 400°F.
2. Boil water salted in a large pan over a medium-high heat.
3. Add sprouts to the pan let boil for 3 minutes.
4. Drain excess water in a colander let dry.

5. Toast the cumin together with the coriander seeds in a small frying pan over a medium heat until fragrant.
6. Grind the toasted seeds with a pinch of sea salt using a mortar.
7. Add the spice mix into a large roasting tray and toss with sprouts.
8. Add onions into the tray with bit of oil.
9. Spread everything in an even layer then, cook for 20 minutes.
10. Return the frying pan to the heat and toast the sesame seeds together with the hazelnuts for 3 minutes.
11. Grind up with the remaining spices, using a mortar.
12. Combine the yoghurt with the tahini.
13. Stir the crushed garlic through with lemon zest juice.
14. Taste the yoghurt and season accordingly.
15. Spread over the base of a large serving platter sprinkled with sumac.
16. Spoon the sprout mix on top of the yoghurt mixture.
17. Sprinkle the ground nuts and seeds over the top.
18. Serve and enjoy with herb leaves scattered on the plate.

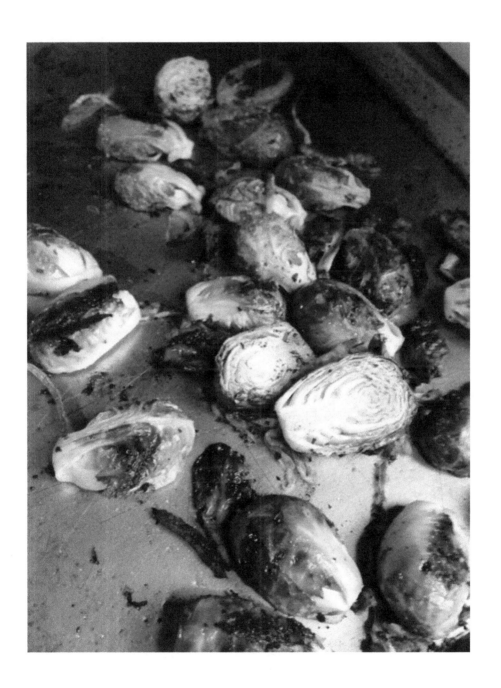

Whole roasted miso aubergine

Ingredients

- 1 tablespoon of tamarind paste
- 4 cloves of garlic
- 3 tablespoons of white sweet miso
- 2 small green chilies
- groundnut oil
- 200g of vine cherry tomatoes
- 3cm piece of ginger
- 4 spring onion
- ½ a bunch of coriander
- 1 lime
- 2 aubergines
- ½ tablespoon of honey

Directions

1. Preheat your oven ready to 350°F.
2. Grate the ginger into a large mortar and pestle, combine together with the garlic, chilies, and a pinch of salt, mix to form a thick paste.
3. Spoon the mixture over the aubergines and massage it into the incisions on the meat.
4. Place the aubergines in a large roasting tray.

5. Dot the cherry tomatoes place into the oven for 40 minutes, turning occasionally.

6. While the aubergines are cooking, trim and finely slice the spring onions and roughly chop the coriander, stalks and all. Add the onions together with the coriander stalks, squeeze over the lime juice to coat and mix well.

7. Combine the tamarind with honey, miso, and water.

8. Remove the roasting tray from the oven after 40 minutes.

9. Raise the heat to high then drizzle the miso glaze over the aubergines.

10. Return back into the oven for more 15 minutes.

11. Remove the stalks from the aubergines and throw away.

12. Chop the flesh in the tray into coarse chunks.

13. Stir in the dressed spring onions.

14. Serve and enjoy.

Roasted brassicas with puy lentil and halloumi

Ingredients

- 1 large bunch of mixed soft herbs
- Olive oil
- 1 heaped teaspoon of baharat
- 2 tablespoons of runny honey
- 4 cloves of garlic
- 250g of puy lentils
- 250g of halloumi cheese
- 1 liter of organic vegetable stock
- 800g of broccoli and cauliflower
- 1 fresh bay leaf
- 2 lemons
- Extra virgin olive oil
- 100g of walnuts

Direction

1. Preheat the oven to 425°F.
2. Spread out the broccoli and cauliflower in a single layer in a roasting tray.
3. Drizzle with olive oil, then sprinkle with Baharat.

4. Season with sea salt and black pepper.

5. Toss in cloves of garlic, spread out in the tray.

6. Roast for 25 minutes.

7. Place lentils in a medium-sized pan.

8. Pour over the hot stock, add the bay leaf.

9. Boil over a medium heat, lower heat let simmer and cook for 30 minutes. Drain and set aside.

10. Mash the garlic until creamy, add lemon juice let season and extra virgin olive oil. Season.

11. Toast the walnuts with the herb leaves. Keep aside.

12. Toss the hot lentils through the garlic dressing, with roasted veggies, herbs and nuts.

13. Pour olive oil into a medium-sized, non-stick frying pan over a medium heat, fry the halloumi till golden.

14. Drizzle with honey and fry for briefly.

15. Serve and enjoy.

Lentil tabbouleh

Ingredients

- 1 lemon
- Extra virgin olive oil
- 1 bunch of spring onions
- 1 large bunch of fresh mint
- 200g of ripe cherry tomatoes
- 200g of lentils
- 1 large bunch of fresh flat-leaf parsley

Directions

1. Cook the lentils in plenty of salted water until tender.
2. Drain any excess water and set aside to cool.
3. Mix the cooled lentils together with the tomatoes, spring onions, herbs, and 4 tablespoons of oil.
4. Add the lemon juice.
5. Season with sea salt and black pepper.
6. Serve and enjoy.

Fresh mango salsa

The Mediterranean mango recipe is quite easy to make is few minutes.

The colorful spicy salad is remarkable delicious especially when served with chips on tacos.

Ingredients

- 1 jalapeño, seeded and minced
- ¼ teaspoon salt, to taste
- 1 medium red bell pepper
- ½ cup of chopped red onion
- 3 ripe mangos
- 1 large lime, juiced
- ¼ cup of packed fresh cilantro leaves

Directions

1. In a serving bowl, combine the prepared mango with bell pepper, onion, cilantro, and jalapeño.
2. Drizzle with the juice of 1 lime.
3. Stir the ingredients together.
4. Season with salt.
5. Serve an enjoy.

Basil pesto salad dressing

Ingredients

- 4 ounces of chopped romaine lettuce
- ½ cup of fresh basil leaves
- Freshly ground pepper
- 4 ounces of fresh spring greens
- 1 clove garlic
- ¼ teaspoon of salt
- 3 tablespoons of raw pine nuts
- Basil pesto dressing
- ½ cup of extra virgin olive oil
- 2 tablespoons of lemon juice

Directions

1. Combine the basil, garlic, and pine nuts in a food blender bowl.
2. Pulse until coarsely chopped.
3. Drizzle in the olive oil, lemon juice, and salt as the machine is running.
4. Season with freshly ground black pepper and blend until smooth.
5. Serve and enjoy.

Simple beet arugula and feta salad with balsamic thyme dressing

Ingredients

- ¼ cup of crumbled feta
- 2 tablespoons of pepitas
- Balsamic thyme dressing
- 2 medium red beets
- Handful of arugula, roughly chopped

Directions

1. Toast the pepitas over a medium heat until fragrant.
2. Transfer to a bowl to cool.
3. Prepare and stack the rounds of beets on top of each other and slice them into long, thin matchsticks.
4. In a medium-sized serving bowl, combine the beets together with the arugula, crumbled feta, and pepitas.
5. Drizzle in enough dressing to coat the salad once tossed.
6. Serve and enjoy.

Peach and avocado green salad

Ingredients

- ½ teaspoon of Dijon mustard
- ½ small red onion
- 1 clove garlic, pressed
- ¼ cup of extra virgin olive oil
- 12 ounces of baby arugula
- ¼ teaspoon of ground black pepper
- ¼ cup of freshly squeezed lemon juice
- ⅔ cup of crumbled mild blue cheese
- 2 medium ripe peaches
- 2 medium ripe avocados
- ¾ teaspoon of kosher salt
- ⅔ cup of unsalted sliced almonds

Directions

1. Place red onion in a small bowl and cover with water.
2. Toast almond in a small skillet over medium-low heat.
3. Let cook until the almonds are fragrant, stirring frequently in 5 minutes.
4. In a small bowl, whisk extra virgin olive oil, lemon juice, Dijon mustard, garlic, kosher salt, and black pepper.
5. Drizzle half of the dressing over the greens, toss.

6. Drain the red onion, scatter over the arugula.
7. Top with the peaches, avocados, almonds and cheese.
8. Serve and enjoy.

Roasted delicata squash, pomegranate, and arugula salad

The roasted delicate squash is a vibrant salad featuring pepitas, feta tossed in a natural balsamic vinaigrette; a perfect choice of Mediterranean Sea diet.

Ingredients

- 1 teaspoon of Dijon mustard
- 2 medium delicata squash
- 2 teaspoons of maple syrup
- 1 ½ tablespoons of balsamic vinegar
- 4 tablespoon of extra virgin olive oil
- Freshly ground black pepper
- Pinch of fine salt
- ¼ teaspoon of fine salt
- 5 ounces of arugula
- Arils from 1 pomegranate
- ⅓ cup of raw pepitas
- 4 ounces of crumbled feta cheese

Directions

1. Preheat your oven ready to 425°F.
2. Drizzle the squash with a tablespoon of olive oil and sprinkle with salt.
3. Bake for 35 minutes in the preheated oven, or until the squash golden, flipping halfway.
4. Toast the pepitas in a medium skillet over medium-low heat, stirring frequently, until fragrant in 5 minutes. Remove.
5. In a small bowl, whisk together the olive oil with balsamic vinegar, maple syrup, Dijon mustard, and salt.
6. Season with black pepper.
7. Combine the arugula, pomegranate, pepitas, crumbled feta, and squash in a large serving bowl.
8. Drizzle in the dressing and toss to combine.
9. Serve and enjoy.

Ginger salad dressing

The ginger salad dressing has a striking flavor drawn from the ginger balanced with sweetness infused with the maple syrup making it a tasty Mediterranean Sea diet recipe.

Ingredients

- ½ cup extra-virgin olive oil
- 2 teaspoons of finely grated fresh ginger
- ½ teaspoon of fine sea salt
- 2 tablespoons of apple cider vinegar
- 20 twists of freshly ground black pepper
- 2 tablespoons of Dijon mustard
- 1 tablespoon of maple syrup

Directions

1. In a small mixing bowl, whisk all of the ingredients listed until completely blended.
2. Taste the seasoning, and adjust accordingly.
3. Serve and enjoy.
4. Any leftovers can be kept refrigerated until consumed.

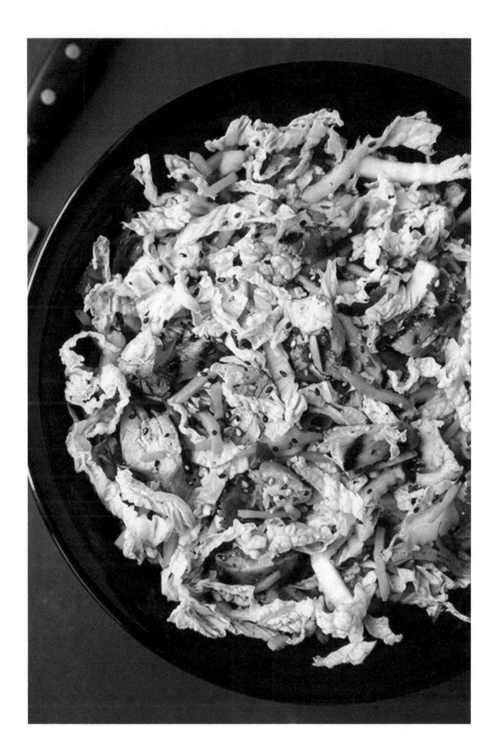

Favorite green salad with apples, cranberries, and pepitas

All the healthy greens you are seeking for are in this Mediterranean Sea diet green salad recipe.

It features apples, pepitas, and cranberries.

Ingredients

- 1 teaspoon of Dijon mustard
- 5 ounces of spring greens salad blend
- 1 ½ tablespoons of apple cider vinegar
- 1 ½ teaspoons of honey
- ¼ teaspoon of fine sea salt
- 1 large apple
- ⅓ cup of dried cranberries
- ¼ cup of pepitas
- Freshly ground black pepper
- 2 ounces of chilled goat cheese
- ¼ cup of extra virgin olive oil

Directions

1. Toast the pepitas over medium heat in a medium-sized skillet, stirring frequently, until golden on the edges.
2. Transfer the pepitas to a small bowl to cool.
3. In a small dish, whisk together the olive oil, honey, vinegar, mustard, and salt until well blended.
4. Season to taste with pepper.
5. Place the greens in a large serving bowl.
6. Top with sliced apple, dried cranberries, and toasted pepitas.
7. Crumble the goat cheese over the salad.
8. Drizzle with enough dressing to lightly coat the leaves once tossed.
9. Serve and enjoy.

Roasted beets and labneh

Do you want to boost blood supply in the body?

If yes, roasted beets is the best Mediterranean Sea diet recipe you can count on to achieve that; served with avocado and herbs.

Ingredients

- 2 cups of fresh basil leaves
- 4 bunches of beets
- 2 tablespoons of red wine vinegar
- ½ teaspoon of red pepper flakes
- ¼ cup of extra virgin olive oil
- 1 teaspoon of red pepper flakes
- Salt and freshly ground black pepper
- 2 cups of labneh
- 1 clove garlic
- 1 teaspoon of kosher salt
- 3 tablespoons of basil vinaigrette
- 2 ripe avocados
- Fresh mint leaves
- Fresh dill leaves
- 3 shallots, roughly chopped

Directions

1. Preheat the oven to 425°F.
2. Line a large baking sheet with parchment paper.
3. Toss wedges of beets with shallots in olive oil.
4. Season with the red pepper flakes, salt and pepper.
5. Transfer the seasoned beets and shallots to the prepared baking sheet
6. Let roast for 50 minutes, until fork tender.
7. Remove, let cool to room temperature.
8. Combine the shallot together with basil, red wine vinegar, garlic, red pepper flakes, olive oil, and salt in a blender.
9. Let blend until very smooth.
10. Season with salt and pepper.
11. Spread the labneh on a large platter
12. Dollop with basil vinaigrette, scatter with the beets and avocado wedges.
13. Then, sprinkle with fresh mint leaves, dill, and flaky salt
14. Serve and enjoy.

Honey mustard Brussels sprout slaw

The Brussels sprouts are neatly shredded and tossed with natural tangy honey mustard, finally dressed with almonds and dried cherries.

It is a perfect choice of Mediterranean Sea diet for vegans.

Ingredients

- 1 tablespoon of Dijon mustard
- 1 pound of Brussels sprouts
- 1 tablespoon of honey
- ⅓ cup of slivered almonds
- ⅓ cup of tart dried cherries
- 1 garlic clove, pressed
- ¼ teaspoon of fine sea salt
- ⅓ cup of shredded Parmesan cheese
- ¼ cup of extra virgin olive oil
- 2 tablespoons of apple cider vinegar

Directions

1. Whisk together the olive oil with vinegar, honey, mustard, and garlic until blended.
2. Toss the shredded sprouts in a medium serving bowl with the almonds, chopped dried fruit, Parmesan, and dressing.
3. Taste, and adjust accordingly.
4. Serve and enjoy immediately.

Layered panzanella salad

Ingredients

- 2 mini cucumbers
- 4 ounces of ciabatta
- 8 ounces of fresh mozzarella
- 2 tablespoons of extra virgin olive oil
- ⅓ cup of roughly chopped fresh basil
- 1 pound of additional tomatoes
- 1 teaspoon fine sea salt
- 3 tablespoons red wine vinegar
- ½ teaspoon dried oregano
- 1 large clove garlic
- 2 tablespoons of thinly sliced Kalamata olives
- Freshly ground black pepper
- ½ small red onion, thinly sliced
- 1 pound of cherry or grape tomatoes

Directions

1. Preheat the oven to 425°F.
2. Slice the bread and place on the baking sheet.
3. Drizzle the cubes with the olive oil and sprinkle with salt, and toss until thoroughly combined.
4. Bake until deeply golden 10 minutes.

5. In a bowl, combine the olive oil together with the vinegar, oregano, garlic, salt, and black pepper. Whisk to combine.

6. Add slice and add onion, or stir into the dressing.

7. Refrigerate in the meantime.

8. Transfer the prepared tomatoes to a large serving platter.

9. Nestle half of the croutons in between the tomatoes, and distribute the rest on top.

10. Place the cucumber rounds with the mozzarella all over the salad.

11. Sprinkle the basil, olives on top, black pepper and dried oregano on top.

12. Serve and enjoy.

Watermelon salad with herbed yogurt sauce

Ingredients

- 1 cup of Greek yogurt
- 2 mini cucumbers
- 1 teaspoon of honey
- Pinch of fine sea salt
- ½ cup of thinly sliced shallot
- 3 tablespoons of sherry vinegar
- ¼ teaspoon of fine sea salt
- 2 tablespoons of extra virgin olive oil
- Small handful fresh mint and basil leaves
- 3 pounds of ripe seedless watermelon
- Flaky sea salt
- Freshly ground black pepper

Directions

1. Start by combining the sliced shallot, vinegar, and ¼ teaspoon salt in a small bowl.
2. Toss to combine, and refrigerate to pickle.
3. Then, in a food processor, combine the yogurt together with the fresh herbs, olive oil, honey, and a pinch of salt.

4. Blend until the herbs are broken into tiny pieces and the sauce is pale green.

5. Swirl the yogurt sauce over the base of the serving platter.

6. Then, scatter the cubed watermelon on top with the cucumber.

7. Organize the pickled shallot on top, and spoon the leftover vinegar over the salad.

8. Drizzle 2 tablespoons olive oil on top.

9. Sprinkle generously with fresh herbs.

10. Season with salt and pepper.

11. Serve and enjoy chilled.

Mediterranean raw squash pasta salad

This is an incredible couscous salad with a bold raw squash flavors.

A typical Mediterranean summer dish delicious enough to keep you hooked on to eating continuously.

Ingredients

- 1 medium zucchini
- ⅓ cup of pitted and thinly sliced Kalamata olives
- 1 ⅓ cup of whole wheat Israeli couscous
- ⅓ cup of pine nuts
- 1 small yellow squash
- ⅓ cup of extra virgin olive oil
- 1 pint of grape tomatoes, quartered
- 4 tablespoons of lemon juice
- ⅓ cup of chopped fresh basil
- 1 large shallot, finely chopped
- 2 cloves garlic, pressed or minced
- 4 ounces of feta cheese
- ½ teaspoon of fine sea salt, to taste
- Freshly ground black pepper

- 1 can of chickpeas, rinsed and drained

Directions

1. Cook the couscous according to package directions.
2. Drain off any excess water.
3. Then toast the pine nut over medium-low heat until turning lightly golden on the sides.
4. Transfer to a bowl to cool.
5. Whisk together the olive oil with lemon juice, shallot, garlic, salt and many twists of black pepper to combined.
6. Add the couscous to the bowl, toss to coat with the dressing.
7. Top the couscous with the toasted pine nuts, feta, olives, chickpeas, tomatoes, zucchini, and squash, and basil. Stir to combine.
8. Season with salt and pepper to taste.
9. Serve and enjoy chilled.

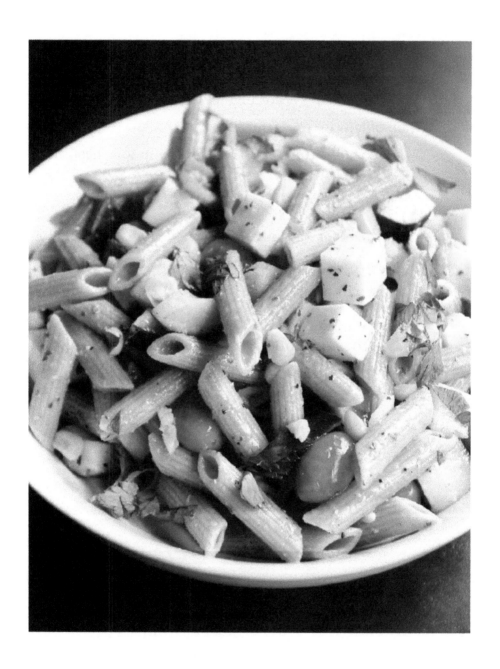

Lightning Source UK Ltd.
Milton Keynes UK
UKHW020714270521
384463UK00001B/52